Easy Dash Diet Meal Prep Beginners Guide

Planning Your Dash Diet Meal Prep

By

David Abhay

Table of Contents

CHAPTER 1

Introduction

1.1 What is the Dash Diet?

The Dash Diet, also known as the Dietary Approaches to Stop Hypertension, is a dietary pattern designed to lower and manage blood pressure levels. It was initially developed by the National Heart, Lung, and Blood Institute (NHLBI) in collaboration with several leading health institutions. However, over time, it has gained popularity as a well-rounded and balanced eating plan for overall health and wellness.

The primary objective of the Dash Diet is to reduce the intake of sodium (salt) while emphasizing the consumption of nutrient-rich foods. It focuses on incorporating whole grains, fruits, vegetables, lean proteins, and low-fat dairy products into the daily meals. By adopting the Dash Diet, individuals can significantly improve their heart health, lower blood pressure, and potentially reduce the risk of other chronic conditions such as stroke, heart disease, and certain types of cancer.

The Dash Diet is supported by extensive research and is considered an evidence-based approach to healthy eating. Several studies have demonstrated its effectiveness in reducing blood pressure levels, even in individuals with hypertension. It offers a balanced and flexible eating plan that can be followed long-term, promoting sustainable lifestyle changes rather than quick-fix solutions.

One of the notable aspects of the Dash Diet is its emphasis on reducing sodium intake. Excessive sodium consumption is known to contribute to high blood pressure. The Dash Diet encourages individuals to limit their sodium intake to 2,300 milligrams (mg) per day, with an ideal target of 1,500 mg for those with hypertension or at risk of developing high blood pressure. This is achieved by minimizing the consumption of processed foods, which tend to be high in sodium, and replacing them with fresh, whole foods prepared at home.

In addition to controlling sodium, the Dash Diet encourages the consumption of other key nutrients that promote heart health. These include potassium, magnesium, calcium, fiber, and protein. Fruits and vegetables are excellent sources of potassium, while low-fat dairy products provide calcium. Whole grains and legumes offer fiber and additional nutrients. Lean proteins, such as poultry, fish, and beans, are recommended over high-fat alternatives.

The Dash Diet is flexible and can be adapted to individual preferences and dietary needs. It does not require strict calorie counting or the elimination of entire food groups. Instead, it focuses on balance and portion control. By following the Dash Diet, individuals learn to make healthier choices and establish sustainable eating habits.

It is important to note that while the Dash Diet is beneficial for many individuals, it is always advisable to consult with a healthcare professional or registered dietitian before making any significant dietary changes, especially if you have specific health conditions or dietary restrictions.

The Dash Diet is a well-researched and effective eating plan designed to reduce blood pressure and improve overall health. It emphasizes the consumption of nutrient-rich foods, while limiting sodium intake. By following the Dash Diet, individuals can promote heart health, manage their blood pressure levels, and make long-term positive changes to their eating habits.

1.2 Benefits of the Dash Diet

The Dash Diet (Dietary Approaches to Stop Hypertension) offers numerous benefits for overall health and well-being. Here are some of the key advantages of following the Dash Diet:

1. Lowered Blood Pressure: One of the primary benefits of the Dash Diet is its ability to effectively lower blood pressure. The emphasis on consuming nutrient-rich foods, such as fruits, vegetables, whole grains, and lean proteins, along with reducing sodium intake, has been shown to have a positive impact on blood pressure levels. Studies have demonstrated that following the Dash Diet can result in

significant reductions in both
systolic and diastolic blood
pressure, making it an effective
dietary approach for individuals
with hypertension or
prehypertension.

2. Heart Health Promotion: The
   Dash Diet is well-known for its
   positive effects on heart health.
   By encouraging the
   consumption of foods that are
   low in saturated fats,
   cholesterol, and sodium, and
   high in heart-healthy nutrients
   such as potassium, magnesium,
   and fiber, the Dash Diet helps
   reduce the risk of
   cardiovascular diseases.
   Lowering blood pressure,
   managing cholesterol levels,
   and promoting overall heart
   health are key factors that

contribute to the diet's cardiovascular benefits.

3. Weight Management: The Dash Diet can also support weight management efforts. The diet emphasizes whole, unprocessed foods that are nutrient-dense and low in calories. By including a variety of fruits, vegetables, lean proteins, and whole grains, the diet promotes satiety and helps individuals feel fuller for longer periods. Additionally, the Dash Diet discourages the consumption of high-calorie, sugary, and processed foods, which can contribute to weight gain. By following the Dash Diet, individuals can establish healthy eating habits that

support long-term weight
management goals.

4. Improved Nutrient Intake: The
Dash Diet encourages the
consumption of a wide range of
nutrient-rich foods, including
fruits, vegetables, whole grains,
lean proteins, and low-fat dairy
products. This variety ensures
that individuals receive a
diverse array of essential
vitamins, minerals,
antioxidants, and dietary fiber.
By focusing on whole foods
rather than processed
alternatives, the Dash Diet
promotes a nutrient-dense
eating pattern that can help
individuals meet their daily
nutritional requirements.

5. Diabetes Management: The
Dash Diet can be beneficial for

individuals with diabetes or those at risk of developing the condition. The diet's emphasis on whole grains, fruits, vegetables, lean proteins, and portion control can help regulate blood sugar levels and improve insulin sensitivity. Additionally, the Dash Diet's emphasis on healthy fats and low sodium intake aligns well with the dietary recommendations for managing diabetes.

6. Flexibility and Long-Term Sustainability: The Dash Diet offers flexibility and can be adapted to personal preferences and cultural dietary habits. It does not restrict or eliminate entire food groups, making it easier to follow and sustain

over the long term. The diet
promotes mindful eating,
portion control, and making
healthier food choices, which
can help individuals establish
sustainable eating habits that
support overall health and well-
being.

It is important to note that individual
results may vary, and the Dash Diet
should be followed in consultation
with a healthcare professional or
registered dietitian, particularly for
individuals with specific health
conditions or dietary restrictions.
However, the overall benefits of the
Dash Diet in promoting heart health,
lowering blood pressure, supporting
weight management, and improving
nutrient intake make it a valuable
dietary approach for many individuals

seeking to improve their overall
health and well-being.

1.3 Getting Started with Meal Prep

Meal prep is a key component of successfully following the Dash Diet and maintaining a healthy eating routine. It involves preparing and portioning meals and snacks in advance to have them readily available throughout the week. Here are some steps to help you get started with meal prep:

1. Set Goals and Plan Ahead: Determine your meal prep goals, whether it's saving time, improving dietary adherence, or promoting portion control. Assess your schedule for the

upcoming week and plan your meals accordingly. Consider the number of meals and snacks you'll need, as well as any specific dietary requirements or preferences.

2. Create a Meal Plan: Develop a meal plan for the week based on the Dash Diet guidelines. Start by identifying the main components of each meal, such as lean proteins, whole grains, fruits, vegetables, and healthy fats. Aim for variety and balance in your meal choices. Plan meals that you enjoy and that fit within your skill level and available time for preparation.

3. Make a Shopping List: Once you have your meal plan, create a detailed shopping list. Take

inventory of the ingredients you already have and note down the items you need to buy. Having a well-organized shopping list will save you time at the grocery store and ensure you have all the necessary ingredients for your meals.

4. Prep Your Kitchen: Before you begin meal prep, ensure that your kitchen is well-equipped and organized. Clean and sanitize your workspace, and gather the necessary kitchen tools and containers for storing your prepped meals. Having the right equipment, such as food storage containers, measuring tools, and sharp knives, will make the meal prep process more efficient.

5. Batch Cooking: Choose a day or time to dedicate to batch cooking. This involves preparing larger quantities of certain ingredients or full meals that can be divided into portions for multiple meals throughout the week. For example, you can cook a large batch of lean proteins like chicken or beans, roast a tray of mixed vegetables, or cook a big pot of whole grains like quinoa or brown rice. Batch cooking saves time and allows you to have pre-prepared components ready for quick assembly during the week.

6. Portion Control: As you prepare your meals, be mindful of portion sizes according to the Dash Diet

recommendations. Use measuring tools, such as measuring cups and food scales, to ensure accurate portioning. Divide the meals into individual or family-sized portions using appropriate containers. Label the containers with the date and contents to stay organized and keep track of freshness.

7. Storage and Freezing: Store your prepped meals and snacks in a refrigerator or freezer based on their shelf life. Foods that will be consumed within a few days can be stored in the refrigerator, while meals that won't be consumed immediately can be portioned and frozen for later use. Ensure that you use airtight containers

to maintain food quality and prevent contamination.

8. Grab-and-Go Snacks: Prepare healthy, Dash Diet-friendly snacks that are easy to grab when you're on the go. Cut up fruits and vegetables into snack-sized portions, portion out nuts or seeds, or make homemade energy balls or granola bars. Having these snacks readily available will help you make healthier choices throughout the day.

9. Stay Organized and Rotate Meals: Keep track of your prepped meals by creating a meal schedule or using a meal planning app. This will help you remember what's available and plan your daily meals accordingly. Additionally, aim

to rotate your meals to avoid
monotony and ensure you're
getting a variety of nutrients.

10. Stay Safe and Reheat Properly:
    When reheating prepped meals,
    follow proper food safety
    guidelines. Ensure that your
    meals are heated to an
    appropriate internal
    temperature to prevent
    foodborne illnesses. Refer to
    recommended reheating times
    and temperatures for different
    types of foods.

By following these steps, you can
streamline your meal preparation
process, save time during the week,
and maintain a healthy eating routine
that aligns with the Dash Diet
guidelines. Meal prep empowers you

to make better food choices and
promotes consistency in your diet,
ultimately supporting your overall
health and well-being.

CHAPTER 2

Understanding the Dash Diet Guidelines

2.1 Dash Diet Food Groups

The Dash Diet emphasizes the consumption of specific food groups that are beneficial for promoting heart health and managing blood pressure. Here are the key food groups in the Dash Diet:

1. Fruits: Fruits are an essential component of the Dash Diet. They are rich in vitamins, minerals, antioxidants, and dietary fiber. The diet

encourages consuming a variety of fruits, both fresh and frozen, to maximize nutrient intake. Examples of fruits commonly included in the Dash Diet are berries, citrus fruits, apples, bananas, melons, and grapes.

2. Vegetables: Vegetables play a crucial role in the Dash Diet as they are low in calories and high in nutrients. Aim to include a wide variety of vegetables in your diet, both raw and cooked. Dark leafy greens, such as spinach, kale, and Swiss chard, are particularly beneficial. Other recommended vegetables include broccoli, carrots, tomatoes, bell peppers, cauliflower, and zucchini.

3. Whole Grains: Whole grains are an important source of fiber, vitamins, and minerals in the Dash Diet. Choose whole grain options over refined grains whenever possible. Include foods such as whole wheat, brown rice, quinoa, barley, oats, and whole grain bread and pasta. These provide sustained energy and contribute to the overall nutritional profile of your meals.

4. Lean Proteins: Lean proteins are a vital part of the Dash Diet. They provide essential amino acids, vitamins, and minerals while being lower in saturated fat compared to high-fat protein sources. Choose lean protein options such as skinless poultry, fish (such as salmon,

trout, and tuna), legumes
(beans, lentils, and peas), and
soy products (tofu, tempeh).
Limit red meat consumption
and opt for lean cuts when
consumed.

5. Low-Fat Dairy Products: The
   Dash Diet includes low-fat
   dairy products as a source of
   calcium and protein. Choose
   low-fat or fat-free options such
   as skim milk, low-fat yogurt,
   and reduced-fat cheese. If you
   have lactose intolerance or
   prefer non-dairy alternatives,
   fortified plant-based milk (soy,
   almond, or oat milk) can be
   used as substitutes.

6. Nuts, Seeds, and Legumes:
   These foods are excellent
   sources of protein, healthy fats,
   fiber, vitamins, and minerals.

Include a variety of nuts and seeds, such as almonds, walnuts, chia seeds, flaxseeds, and sunflower seeds. Legumes, including beans, lentils, chickpeas, and peas, are also recommended as they provide plant-based protein and fiber.

7. Healthy Fats: The Dash Diet encourages the consumption of healthy fats while limiting saturated and trans fats. Include sources of monounsaturated and polyunsaturated fats, such as olive oil, avocado, nuts, and seeds. These fats have been associated with positive effects on heart health when consumed in moderation.

8. Sodium Restrictions: The Dash Diet emphasizes reducing sodium intake to help lower

blood pressure. Limiting processed foods, which are often high in sodium, is essential. Instead, use herbs, spices, and salt-free seasonings to add flavor to meals. It is important to read food labels carefully and choose lower sodium options whenever possible.

Remember that portion sizes and overall calorie intake are also important factors to consider within the Dash Diet guidelines. The recommended daily caloric intake varies depending on factors such as age, sex, activity level, and individual health goals.

By incorporating these food groups into your daily meals, you can create a balanced and nutritious eating pattern that aligns with the Dash Diet guidelines. These food groups provide a wide range of essential nutrients while promoting heart health and helping to manage blood pressure levels.

2.2 Sodium Intake Recommendations

The Dash Diet places a strong emphasis on reducing sodium intake to help lower and manage blood pressure levels. Excessive sodium consumption has been linked to high blood pressure, a major risk factor for heart disease and stroke. Here are the sodium intake recommendations in the Dash Diet:

1. General Sodium Intake Recommendation: The Dash Diet recommends limiting

sodium intake to 2,300 milligrams (mg) per day. This is the general guideline for healthy individuals without hypertension or other medical conditions. It's important to note that the average sodium intake in many Western diets far exceeds this recommendation.

2. Lower Sodium Intake Recommendation: For individuals who already have high blood pressure or are at risk of developing it, a lower sodium intake target of 1,500 mg per day is recommended. This lower sodium level is associated with greater reductions in blood pressure and improved cardiovascular health.

3. Sodium Reduction Strategies:
   To achieve these sodium intake
   recommendations, the Dash
   Diet encourages adopting
   strategies to reduce sodium
   consumption:

a. Read Food Labels: Pay close
attention to the sodium content listed
on food labels. Look for lower-
sodium options or choose products
labeled as "low sodium" or "no added
salt."

b. Limit Processed Foods: Many
processed and packaged foods, such
as canned soups, deli meats, snacks,
and condiments, are high in sodium.
Minimize their consumption and opt
for fresh, whole foods prepared at
home whenever possible.

c. Cook at Home: By preparing meals
from scratch, you have control over

the ingredients and sodium content. Use fresh herbs, spices, lemon juice, vinegar, and salt-free seasonings to enhance the flavors of your dishes instead of relying on added salt.

d. Reduce Salt During Cooking: Use less salt when cooking. Experiment with herbs, spices, and other flavorings to enhance the taste of your meals.

e. Be Mindful of Hidden Sodium: Be aware that sodium can be present in unexpected places, such as sauces, dressings, and even certain medications. Check labels and choose low-sodium alternatives.

f. Limit Fast Food and Restaurant Meals: These meals often contain high amounts of sodium due to added salt and other sodium-rich ingredients. Opt for healthier choices when dining out, and request meals to be prepared with less or no added salt.

g. Gradual Reduction: If you are accustomed to a high-sodium diet, aim to gradually reduce your sodium intake over time. This allows your taste buds to adjust, and you may find that you become more sensitive to the taste of salt.

It's important to note that sodium reduction should be implemented in consultation with a healthcare professional, particularly if you have specific health conditions or dietary restrictions. They can provide personalized recommendations based on your individual needs.

By following the sodium intake recommendations and implementing strategies to reduce sodium in your diet, you can align your eating habits with the Dash Diet and support better blood pressure management and overall cardiovascular health.

2.3 Daily Calorie Goals

The Dash Diet does not prescribe specific calorie goals, as calorie needs vary based on factors such as age, sex, weight, height, activity level, and individual health goals. However, the Dash Diet encourages portion control and balanced meals to support a healthy weight and overall well-being. Here are some general principles to consider when determining your calorie goals within the context of the Dash Diet:

1. Assess Your Energy Needs: Start by estimating your daily energy needs based on factors such as your basal metabolic rate (BMR), which is the

number of calories your body needs to perform basic functions at rest, and your activity level. Various online calculators and equations can provide estimates, but consulting with a registered dietitian or healthcare professional may offer a more accurate assessment tailored to your specific needs.

2. Aim for a Healthy Weight: If you are looking to maintain a healthy weight, your daily calorie intake should match your energy expenditure. This means consuming an amount of calories that balances your energy intake with the energy you burn through physical activity and bodily functions. This balance is important for

weight maintenance and overall health.

3. Calorie Deficit for Weight Loss: If your goal is weight loss, creating a calorie deficit is necessary. A calorie deficit occurs when you consume fewer calories than your body needs. However, it's essential to create a moderate deficit that allows for sustainable weight loss and supports overall health. Aiming for a deficit of 500-1,000 calories per day is generally considered safe and effective for gradual and sustainable weight loss of 1-2 pounds per week.

4. Individualized Approach: It is crucial to remember that individual needs can vary significantly. Factors such as

genetics, metabolism, and body composition play a role in determining optimal calorie intake. Consulting with a registered dietitian can help determine the most appropriate calorie goals for your unique situation and goals.

5. Balanced Macronutrient Distribution: Regardless of calorie goals, the Dash Diet emphasizes a balanced distribution of macronutrients. This includes consuming a variety of fruits, vegetables, whole grains, lean proteins, and healthy fats in appropriate portions. These foods provide essential nutrients while promoting satiety and overall health.

6. Adjustments for Physical
    Activity: If you are physically
    active, your calorie needs may
    be higher to support your
    activity level. Consider your
    exercise routine and adjust your
    calorie intake accordingly to
    ensure you have enough energy
    for your workouts and
    recovery.

The Dash Diet focuses on overall dietary patterns and food choices rather than strict calorie counting. It promotes a well-balanced approach to eating, incorporating nutrient-rich foods while reducing sodium and unhealthy fats. Individualized guidance from a registered dietitian can provide personalized recommendations tailored to your needs and goals.

It is always important to consult with
a healthcare professional or registered
dietitian before making significant
changes to your calorie intake or
embarking on a weight loss journey to
ensure that your approach is safe and
suitable for your individual
circumstances.

CHAPTER 3

Essential Kitchen Tools for Dash Diet Meal Prep

3.1 Meal Prep Containers

When it comes to meal prepping for the Dash Diet, having the right containers is essential for storing and portioning your prepared meals. Here are some types of meal prep containers that can be helpful for your Dash Diet meal prep:

1. BPA-Free Plastic Containers: These containers are lightweight, durable, and come in various sizes and shapes. Look for BPA-free options to

ensure the containers are safe for food storage. They are often microwave-safe and dishwasher-safe, making reheating and cleaning convenient. Choose containers with tight-fitting lids to prevent leaks and maintain the freshness of your meals.

2. Glass Containers: Glass containers are a popular choice for meal prep as they are non-toxic, do not absorb odors or stains, and can be reheated in the oven or microwave. They are also a sustainable option since they can be reused for a long time. Look for glass containers with snap-on or locking lids to keep your meals secure during storage and transportation.

3. Sectioned Containers:
    Sectioned or
    compartmentalized containers
    are particularly useful for
    separating different
    components of your meals.
    These containers have multiple
    compartments, allowing you to
    portion out your proteins,
    grains, vegetables, and sauces
    separately. They are great for
    maintaining the integrity of
    each food group and preventing
    them from mixing together.

4. Mason Jars: Mason jars are
    versatile and can be used for
    various purposes in meal prep.
    They are great for storing
    salads, overnight oats, parfaits,
    or layered snacks. The clear
    glass allows you to see the
    layers and create visually

appealing meals. Mason jars
with screw-on lids are preferred
for easy sealing and
transportation.

5. Silicone Reusable Bags: These
    eco-friendly alternatives to
    plastic bags are ideal for storing
    individual servings of snacks,
    sliced fruits, or portioned
    ingredients. Silicone bags are
    durable, leak-proof, and can be
    washed and reused, reducing
    waste.

6. Freezer-Safe Containers: If you
    plan on freezing portions of
    your meals, make sure to use
    containers specifically designed
    for freezer storage. These
    containers are made of
    materials that can withstand
    low temperatures without
    cracking or breaking. Look for

containers that are both freezer-safe and microwave-safe for convenient reheating.

7. Portion-Controlled Containers: To help with portion control, consider using containers that have built-in portion compartments or markings. These containers have pre-determined sections to guide you in portioning your proteins, grains, and vegetables according to the Dash Diet guidelines.

Remember to choose containers that are appropriate for your needs, including the number of meals you plan to prep, the type of foods you'll be storing, and your preferred method of reheating. It's also helpful to have a variety of container sizes to accommodate different portion sizes and meal types.

Regardless of the containers you choose, make sure they are food-grade, easy to clean, and seal properly to maintain the freshness and integrity of your meals. Investing in quality meal prep containers will make your Dash Diet meal prep more organized, convenient, and enjoyable.

3.2 Kitchen Utensils

Having the right kitchen utensils can make your Dash Diet meal prep more efficient and enjoyable. Here are some essential kitchen utensils that can help you with your meal preparation:

1. Chef's Knife: A good-quality chef's knife is an essential tool

for cutting, chopping, and slicing fruits, vegetables, and proteins. Look for a sharp, durable knife that feels comfortable in your hand.

2. Cutting Board: Invest in a sturdy cutting board that is large enough to accommodate various ingredients. opt for a cutting board made of materials such as bamboo, wood, or plastic, depending on your preference.

3. Measuring Cups and Spoons: Accurate measurement of ingredients is important for portion control and following recipes. Have a set of measuring cups and spoons to measure liquids, dry ingredients, and spices.

4. Mixing Bowls: Having a few
    different-sized mixing bowls
    can be helpful for combining
    ingredients, marinating
    proteins, tossing salads, and
    mixing dressings or sauces.

5. Whisk: A whisk is useful for
    blending ingredients, beating
    eggs, and emulsifying dressings
    or sauces. Look for a whisk
    with a comfortable handle and
    sturdy wires.

6. Spatulas: Silicone or rubber
    spatulas are versatile tools for
    mixing, scraping, and folding
    ingredients. They are gentle on
    cookware and ideal for non-
    stick pans.

7. Tongs: Tongs are useful for
    flipping meats, tossing salads,
    and serving vegetables. Choose

tongs with a good grip and locking mechanism for easy storage.

8. Vegetable Peeler: A vegetable peeler makes peeling fruits and vegetables quick and efficient. Look for a peeler with a sharp blade and comfortable handle.

9. Grater/Zester: A grater or zester is handy for grating cheese, zesting citrus fruits, or grating vegetables like carrots. Look for a grater with different-sized grating surfaces.

10. Oven-Safe Baking Dish or Sheet Pan: If you plan to roast or bake meals as part of your Dash Diet meal prep, having an oven-safe baking dish or sheet pan is essential. Choose one

that is of high quality and suitable for your oven.

11. Blender or Food Processor: A blender or food processor can be helpful for making smoothies, pureeing soups, or preparing sauces and dressings. Look for a model with different speed settings and a strong motor.

12. Salad Spinner: A salad spinner is useful for washing and drying greens and vegetables, ensuring they are clean and ready to use in your salads or meals.

3.3 Pantry Staples

To make your Dash Diet meal prep easier and more convenient, it's helpful to keep your pantry stocked with essential staples. Here are some pantry staples that are commonly used in Dash Diet recipes:

1. Whole Grains: Keep a variety of whole grains on hand, such as brown rice, quinoa, whole wheat pasta, whole grain bread, oats, and barley. These provide the foundation for many Dash Diet meals.

2. Canned Beans and Legumes: Stock up on canned beans, such as black beans, kidney beans, chickpeas, and lentils. They are excellent sources of plant-based protein and fiber.

3. Canned Tomatoes: Canned tomatoes, including diced, crushed, or pureed varieties, are

versatile for making sauces, soups, and stews.

4. Low-Sodium Broth or Stock: Having low-sodium vegetable, chicken, or beef broth or stock on hand can enhance the flavors of your dishes without adding excessive sodium.

5. Olive Oil: Choose extra-virgin olive oil as your primary cooking oil. It is a heart-healthy option for sautéing, roasting, and dressing salads.

6. Herbs and Spices: Keep a well-stocked selection of herbs and spices to add flavor to your meals without relying on excessive salt. Include staples like garlic powder, onion powder, dried herbs (such as oregano, basil, thyme, and

rosemary), and spices (such as cumin, paprika, turmeric, and cinnamon).

7. Vinegars: Keep a variety of vinegars on hand, such as balsamic vinegar, red wine vinegar, apple cider vinegar, and white vinegar. They can be used to create flavorful dressings, marinades, and sauces.

8. Low-Sodium Soy Sauce or Tamari: If you enjoy Asian flavors, opt for low-sodium soy sauce or tamari to season your dishes while minimizing sodium content.

9. Nuts and Seeds: Store a variety of nuts and seeds, such as almonds, walnuts, chia seeds, flaxseeds, and sunflower seeds.

They can be used as toppings
for salads, yogurts, or
incorporated into recipes.

10. Nut Butter: Choose natural nut
    butter, such as almond butter or
    peanut butter, without added
    sugars or excessive sodium. It
    can be used as a spread, added
    to smoothies, or used as an
    ingredient in sauces and
    dressings.

11. Dried Fruits: Have dried fruits,
    like raisins, cranberries, or
    apricots, on hand to add natural
    sweetness to dishes, oatmeal, or
    trail mix.

12. Low-Sodium Seasonings and
    Condiments: Opt for low-
    sodium seasonings, such as
    herb blends or salt-free
    seasoning mixes, to enhance

the flavors of your meals. Also, have condiments like mustard, hot sauce, and salsa on hand to add variety and taste to your dishes.

Keeping these pantry staples stocked will provide you with a solid foundation for preparing flavorful and nutritious Dash Diet meals. Regularly check the expiration dates and replenish items as needed to ensure freshness and quality.

CHAPTER 4

Planning Your Dash Diet Meal Prep

4.1 Setting Goals and Creating a Meal Plan

Setting clear goals and creating a meal plan are crucial steps in successful Dash Diet meal prep. By defining your objectives and planning ahead, you can ensure that your meals align with the Dash Diet guidelines and meet your individual needs. Here's a step-by-step guide:

1. Define Your Goals: Start by determining your goals for following the Dash Diet. Are you looking to manage or lower

your blood pressure, improve heart health, lose weight, or simply adopt a healthier eating pattern? Identifying your goals will help you tailor your meal plan accordingly.

2. Assess Your Current Eating Habits: Take an honest look at your current eating habits. Evaluate the types of foods you typically consume and areas where improvements can be made. Consider any challenges or barriers that may impact your ability to follow the Dash Diet consistently.

3. Understand Dash Diet Guidelines: Familiarize yourself with the Dash Diet guidelines. Understand the recommended food groups, portion sizes, and restrictions,

such as limiting sodium intake.
Refer to reliable sources, such
as reputable websites or books,
to gain a comprehensive
understanding of the diet's
principles.

4. Determine Calorie Needs:
    Estimate your daily calorie
    needs based on your age, sex,
    weight, height, activity level,
    and goals. Online calculators or
    consulting with a registered
    dietitian can help provide a
    personalized estimation. While
    the Dash Diet does not focus on
    strict calorie counting, having a
    general idea of your caloric
    requirements can guide your
    meal planning.

5. Identify Meal and Snack
    Frequencies: Decide how many
    meals and snacks you plan to

have each day. The Dash Diet generally recommends three meals and one to two snacks, but you can adjust this based on your personal preference and schedule.

6. Plan Your Meals: Begin creating a meal plan for the week based on the Dash Diet guidelines and your goals. Ensure that each meal includes a balance of the recommended food groups, including fruits, vegetables, whole grains, lean proteins, low-fat dairy products, and healthy fats. Consider the specific Dash Diet recommendations for each food group, such as portion sizes and sodium limitations.

7. Consider Batch Cooking: Incorporate batch cooking into

your meal plan to save time and ensure you have prepared components readily available. Identify meals that can be made in larger quantities and portioned out for future use. This can include cooking grains, roasting vegetables, or preparing proteins in advance.

8. Variety and Flexibility: Aim for variety in your meal plan to prevent monotony and ensure a wide range of nutrients. Consider the inclusion of different flavors, textures, and cooking methods to make your meals enjoyable. Flexibility is also important, allowing for adjustments based on seasonal produce availability, preferences, and changing schedules.

9. Plan for Leftovers: Utilize leftovers effectively in your meal plan. Consider how you can repurpose leftovers into new meals or incorporate them as components in other dishes. This reduces food waste and simplifies your meal prep process.

10. Track and Assess: Consider using a meal planning app, a spreadsheet, or a simple pen and paper to track your meal plan. This helps you stay organized, ensures you have the necessary ingredients, and allows you to assess your adherence to the Dash Diet guidelines.

4.2 Grocery Shopping for Dash Diet Meal Prep

After creating your meal plan, it's time to make a grocery shopping list that aligns with the Dash Diet principles. Here's a guide to help you with your Dash Diet grocery shopping:

1. Review Your Meal Plan: Refer to your meal plan and identify the ingredients needed for each meal and snack. Take note of quantities, including fresh produce, proteins, grains, dairy products, and pantry staples.

2. Focus on Fresh Produce: Allocate a significant portion of your grocery list to fresh fruits and vegetables. Choose a variety of colorful options to ensure a wide range of

nutrients. opt for seasonal produce when possible, for better flavor and affordability.

3. Select Lean Proteins: Include lean protein sources on your list, such as skinless poultry, fish, beans, lentils, tofu, and low-fat dairy products. Consider the portion sizes and quantities needed for your meals and snacks throughout the week.

4. Whole Grains and Legumes: Add whole grains, such as quinoa, brown rice, whole wheat bread, and whole grain pasta, to your list. Include legumes like chickpeas, black beans, and lentils for additional protein and fiber.

5. Low-Sodium Options: Pay
    attention to sodium content
    when selecting canned goods,
    such as beans, tomatoes, and
    broths. Look for low-sodium or
    no-salt-added versions to align
    with the Dash Diet's sodium
    restrictions.

6. Healthy Fats: Include sources
    of healthy fats on your list,
    such as extra-virgin olive oil,
    nuts, seeds, and avocados.
    These can be used for cooking,
    as toppings, or for making
    homemade salad dressings.

7. Spices, Herbs, and Seasonings:
    Stock up on a variety of spices,
    herbs, and salt-free seasonings
    to add flavor to your meals
    without relying on excessive
    sodium. Consider options like
    garlic powder, onion powder,

oregano, basil, cumin, turmeric, and cinnamon.

8. Non-Perishable Pantry Staples: Check your pantry for items like whole grain oats, whole wheat flour, low-sodium soy sauce or tamari, vinegar, nut butter, dried fruits, and low-sodium seasonings. Add these items to your shopping list if needed.

9. Review and Organize: Once your shopping list is complete, review it to ensure you have all the necessary ingredients for your meal plan. Organize the list according to sections in the grocery store to make your shopping trip more efficient.

10. Stick to the List: While at the grocery store, stay focused on

your shopping list and avoid impulse purchases. Be mindful of labels and choose items that align with the Dash Diet guidelines, such as low-sodium options and nutrient-dense foods.

By setting goals, creating a meal plan, and making a well-organized grocery shopping list, you can ensure that your Dash Diet meal prep aligns with your objectives and supports your overall health and well-being.

4.3 Batch Cooking and Prepping in Advance

Batch cooking and prepping in advance are key strategies for successful Dash Diet meal prep. By dedicating some time to prepare and cook larger quantities of food, you can save time throughout the week and ensure that healthy meals are readily available. Here's how to incorporate batch cooking and prepping into your Dash Diet meal prep routine:

1. Select Batch-Friendly Recipes: Choose recipes that are suitable for batch cooking and can be easily divided into portions for multiple meals. Recipes that include lean proteins, whole grains, and vegetables are ideal. Examples include chili, soups, stews, casseroles, roasted vegetables, and grain-based salads.

2. Plan Your Batch Cooking Day: Designate a specific day or time during the week for your batch cooking session. This will

depend on your schedule and personal preferences. Many people find it convenient to do batch cooking on weekends when they have more free time.

3. Create a Cooking Schedule: Prioritize your recipes based on cooking times and oven or stovetop availability. Make a schedule to ensure that you optimize your time and multitask effectively. For example, while a casserole is baking in the oven, you can prepare another dish on the stovetop.

4. Cook Proteins in Bulk: Prepare a larger quantity of lean proteins, such as chicken breasts, turkey, lean beef, or fish, during your batch cooking session. Season and cook them

according to your recipe or simply bake or grill them plain for versatility. Once cooked, portion out the proteins into meal-sized portions and refrigerate or freeze them for later use.

5. Cook Whole Grains and Beans: Cook a batch of whole grains like quinoa, brown rice, or whole wheat pasta. Prepare beans or legumes like lentils, chickpeas, or black beans. These can be used as a base for salads, side dishes, or added to soups and stews throughout the week.

6. Roast or Steam Vegetables: Roast or steam a variety of vegetables during your batch cooking session. Choose vegetables like broccoli,

cauliflower, carrots, bell peppers, or Brussels sprouts. Portion them out into containers or ziplock bags and refrigerate or freeze them for easy meal assembly later on.

7. Portion and Store: Once your batch cooking is complete, portion out the cooked components into meal-sized containers. Label each container with the date and contents to stay organized. Refrigerate the portions you plan to consume within a few days and freeze the rest for longer-term storage. Ensure that you use airtight containers to maintain freshness and prevent freezer burn.

8. Meal Assembly: When it's time to enjoy your prepped meals,

simply take out the desired components from the refrigerator or freezer and assemble your meals. Combine proteins, grains, and vegetables in appropriate portions, and add flavor with herbs, spices, and dressings. Add fresh ingredients, such as chopped tomatoes, cucumbers, or herbs, to enhance the flavors and textures.

9. Use in Different Recipes: Don't be afraid to get creative and use your batch-cooked components in various recipes throughout the week. For example, roasted vegetables can be added to salads, grain bowls, or wraps. Cooked proteins can be incorporated into stir-fries, salads, or sandwiches.

10. Reheat Properly: When reheating your prepped meals, ensure that they are heated to a safe internal temperature to prevent foodborne illnesses. Follow recommended reheating times and temperatures for different types of foods. Microwave, stovetop, or oven reheating methods can be used based on convenience and personal preference.

By incorporating batch cooking and prepping in advance into your Dash Diet meal prep routine, you can save time, ensure meal variety, and have healthy options readily available throughout the week. It allows you to enjoy the benefits of the Dash Diet while minimizing the time spent on daily meal preparation.

CHAPTER 5

Breakfast Ideas and Recipes

5.1 Dash Diet Breakfast Guidelines

Breakfast is an important meal that sets the tone for the rest of the day. When following the Dash Diet, it's important to choose breakfast options that align with the guidelines and provide a balanced combination of nutrients. Here are some Dash Diet breakfast guidelines to keep in mind:

1. Include Whole Grains: Choose whole grain options for your breakfast to provide fiber, vitamins, and minerals. Opt for

whole wheat bread, oatmeal, whole grain cereals, or quinoa as a base for your breakfast dishes.

2. Add Fruits and Vegetables: Incorporate fruits and vegetables into your breakfast to increase nutrient content and add flavor. Enjoy a side of fresh berries, sliced fruit, or add vegetables like spinach, bell peppers, or tomatoes to omelets or breakfast wraps.

3. Include Lean Proteins: Include lean sources of protein in your breakfast to help you feel full and satisfied. Consider options such as low-fat dairy products like Greek yogurt or cottage cheese, eggs, egg whites, lean turkey or chicken sausage, or legumes like beans or lentils.

4. Healthy Fats: Incorporate small amounts of healthy fats into your breakfast for flavor and satiety. Options include adding a tablespoon of nut butter to your toast or oatmeal, sprinkling chopped nuts or seeds on your yogurt or cereal, or drizzling extra-virgin olive oil over a vegetable omelet.

5. Watch Sodium Intake: Be mindful of the sodium content in your breakfast choices. opt for low-sodium or no-salt-added versions of packaged foods like cereals, bread, and deli meats. Use herbs, spices, and salt-free seasonings to add flavor instead of relying on added salt.

6. Portion Control: Pay attention to portion sizes to ensure a

balanced breakfast. Use measuring cups or a food scale to measure appropriate portions of grains, proteins, and fats. This will help you achieve the recommended serving sizes and maintain calorie control.

7. Hydration: Don't forget to include a hydrating beverage as part of your breakfast routine. Water, herbal tea, or a small glass of 100% fruit juice can be refreshing options.

The Dash Diet is flexible, and you can adapt breakfast options to suit your preferences and dietary needs. Use these guidelines as a starting point to create a balanced and nutritious breakfast that aligns with the Dash Diet principles.

5.2 Easy Dash Diet Breakfast Recipes

Here are a few easy and delicious Dash Diet breakfast recipes to inspire your morning routine:

1. Veggie Omelet: Ingredients:

   - 2 eggs

   - 1/4 cup diced vegetables (bell peppers, onions, spinach, tomatoes)

   - 1 tablespoon shredded low-fat cheese

   - Salt-free seasoning to taste

   - 1 teaspoon extra-virgin olive oil

Instructions:

   - In a bowl, whisk the eggs until well beaten. Add salt-free seasoning.

- Heat olive oil in a non-stick skillet over medium heat.

- Add the diced vegetables and sauté until slightly softened.

- Pour the beaten eggs over the vegetables and cook until the bottom is set.

- Sprinkle the shredded cheese over one half of the omelet and fold the other half over the top.

- Cook for another minute until the cheese melts.

- Serve with a side of whole wheat toast or fresh fruit.

2. Overnight Chia Pudding:
Ingredients:

- 2 tablespoons chia seeds

- 1/2 cup low-fat milk or unsweetened almond milk

- 1/4 teaspoon vanilla extract

- 1 tablespoon honey or maple syrup

- Fresh berries or sliced fruit for topping

Instructions:

- In a jar or container, combine chia seeds, milk, vanilla extract, and sweetener.

- Stir well to combine and ensure the chia seeds are evenly distributed.

- Cover and refrigerate overnight or for at least 4 hours.

- Before serving, stir the mixture again to break up any clumps.

- Top with fresh berries or sliced fruit.

- Enjoy as is or add a sprinkle of chopped nuts or seeds for added crunch.

3. Greek Yogurt Parfait:
   Ingredients:

- 1/2 cup plain Greek yogurt

- 1/4 cup granola (choose a low-sugar and whole grain option)

- 1/4 cup mixed fresh berries (such as strawberries, blueberries, raspberries)

- 1 tablespoon honey or maple syrup (optional)

Instructions:

- In a glass or bowl, layer half of the Greek yogurt.

- Sprinkle half of the granola over the yogurt layer.

- Add half of the mixed berries
  on top.

- Repeat the layers with the
  remaining ingredients.

- Drizzle with honey or maple
  syrup if desired.

- Enjoy immediately or
  refrigerate until ready to eat.

4. Whole Grain Toast with
   Avocado and Egg: Ingredients:

- 1 slice whole grain bread,
  toasted

- 1/4 ripe avocado, mashed

- 1 poached or soft-boiled egg

- Salt-free seasoning or herbs of
  choice (such as black pepper,
  paprika, or chili flakes)

Instructions:

- Spread the mashed avocado evenly on the toasted bread slice.

- Place the poached or soft-boiled egg on top.

- Sprinkle with salt-free seasoning or herbs.

- Serve with a side of fresh fruit or a small handful of baby carrots.

These recipes are just a starting point, and you can customize them to suit your taste preferences and ingredient availability. Remember to adjust portion sizes and ingredient quantities according to your specific calorie needs and goals.

CHAPTER 6

Lunch Ideas and Recipes

6.1 Dash Diet Lunch Guidelines

Lunchtime provides an opportunity to refuel and nourish your body with a balanced meal. When following the Dash Diet, it's important to make nutritious choices that align with the guidelines. Here are some Dash Diet lunch guidelines to consider:

1. Incorporate Fruits and Vegetables: Include a variety of colorful fruits and vegetables in your lunch to maximize nutrient intake. This can be

done through salads, vegetable-based soups, stir-fries, or by adding sliced vegetables to sandwiches or wraps.

2. Choose Lean Proteins: Opt for lean protein sources to promote satiety and support muscle health. This can include skinless poultry, fish, beans, lentils, tofu, or low-fat dairy products like yogurt or cottage cheese. Aim for portion sizes that meet your protein needs.

3. Emphasize Whole Grains: Select whole grain options for your lunch to provide fiber, vitamins, and minerals. Whole grain bread, whole wheat pasta, brown rice, quinoa, or whole grain wraps can be used as a base for your lunch meals.

4. Include Healthy Fats:
    Incorporate small amounts of
    healthy fats into your lunch for
    flavor and satiety. This can be
    achieved through ingredients
    like nuts, seeds, avocado, or a
    drizzle of extra-virgin olive oil
    in salads or dressings.

5. Watch Sodium Intake: Be
    mindful of the sodium content
    in your lunch choices. Limit the
    use of high-sodium condiments
    and processed foods. Instead,
    opt for homemade dressings
    and seasonings with herbs,
    spices, and salt-free blends.

6. Control Portion Sizes: Pay
    attention to portion control to
    ensure a balanced lunch. Use
    measuring cups or a food scale
    to measure appropriate portions
    of grains, proteins, and fats.

This helps maintain calorie control and adherence to the Dash Diet guidelines.

7. Hydration: Accompany your lunch with a hydrating beverage, such as water, herbal tea, or infused water with sliced fruits or herbs. Limit sugary drinks and opt for healthier options.

6.2 Simple Dash Diet Lunch Recipes

Here are a few simple and delicious Dash Diet lunch recipes to inspire your midday meals:

1. Mediterranean Chickpea Salad: Ingredients:

- 1 can chickpeas, drained and rinsed

- 1 cup cherry tomatoes, halved

- 1 cucumber, diced

- 1/4 red onion, thinly sliced

- 1/4 cup chopped Kalamata olives

- 2 tablespoons crumbled feta cheese

- Fresh parsley, chopped

- Juice of 1 lemon

- 2 tablespoons extra-virgin olive oil

- Salt-free seasoning to taste

Instructions:

- In a large bowl, combine chickpeas, cherry tomatoes,

cucumber, red onion, Kalamata
olives, and feta cheese.

- In a small bowl, whisk together
  lemon juice, olive oil, and salt-
  free seasoning.

- Pour the dressing over the salad
  and toss to coat.

- Sprinkle with fresh parsley
  before serving.

2. Turkey and Vegetable Wrap:
   Ingredients:

- 1 whole grain wrap or tortilla

- 4 ounces sliced turkey breast

- 1/4 avocado, sliced

- 1/4 cup sliced bell peppers

- 1/4 cup shredded lettuce

- 1 tablespoon hummus

- Salt-free seasoning or herbs of choice

Instructions:

- Lay the whole grain wrap or tortilla flat.

- Spread hummus evenly over the wrap.

- Layer sliced turkey, avocado, bell peppers, and shredded lettuce on top.

- Sprinkle with salt-free seasoning or herbs.

- Roll up the wrap tightly and slice in half if desired.

3. Quinoa and Vegetable Stir-Fry: Ingredients:

- 1 cup cooked quinoa

- 1 tablespoon extra-virgin olive oil

- 1 cup mixed vegetables (such as broccoli florets, bell peppers, carrots, snap peas)

- 2 cloves garlic, minced

- 2 tablespoons low-sodium soy sauce or tamari

- Salt-free seasoning to taste

- Optional: cooked chicken breast or tofu for added protein

Instructions:

- Heat olive oil in a large skillet or wok over medium-high heat.

- Add the minced garlic and sauté for 1 minute until fragrant.

- Add the mixed vegetables and stir-fry until crisp-tender.

- Stir in the cooked quinoa and cooked chicken breast or tofu if using.

- Drizzle low-sodium soy sauce or tamari over the mixture and sprinkle with salt-free seasoning.

- Stir-fry for another 2-3 minutes until everything is heated through.

- Adjust seasoning if needed and serve hot.

4. Greek Salad with Grilled Chicken: Ingredients:

- 4 ounces grilled chicken breast, sliced

- 2 cups mixed salad greens

- 1/4 cup cherry tomatoes, halved

- 1/4 cucumber, sliced

- 2 tablespoons sliced red onion

- 2 tablespoons crumbled feta cheese

- Kalamata olives (optional)

- Lemon juice for dressing

- 1 teaspoon extra-virgin olive oil

- Salt-free seasoning to taste

Instructions:

- In a bowl, combine mixed salad greens, cherry tomatoes, cucumber, red onion, feta cheese, and Kalamata olives if desired.

- Drizzle with lemon juice and olive oil.

- Sprinkle with salt-free
  seasoning and toss to combine.

- Top the salad with sliced
  grilled chicken breast.

- Serve immediately.

These recipes can be customized according to your taste preferences and dietary needs. Adjust portion sizes and ingredient quantities to meet your specific calorie goals. Enjoy these simple and nutritious lunch options as part of your Dash Diet meal plan.

CHAPTER 7

Dinner Ideas and Recipes

7.1 Dash Diet Dinner Guidelines

Dinner is an important meal that allows you to wind down and refuel after a long day. When following the Dash Diet, it's important to choose nutritious options that align with the guidelines. Here are some Dash Diet dinner guidelines to keep in mind:

1. Balance Your Plate: Aim for a well-balanced dinner that includes a variety of food groups. Include lean proteins, whole grains, vegetables, and

healthy fats to create a satisfying and nutritious meal.

2. Lean Proteins: Choose lean sources of protein for your dinner, such as skinless poultry, fish, beans, lentils, tofu, or lean cuts of meat. These options provide essential amino acids and support muscle health.

3. Whole Grains: Incorporate whole grains into your dinner to provide fiber, vitamins, and minerals. Options include brown rice, quinoa, whole wheat pasta, barley, or whole grain bread.

4. Plenty of Vegetables: Fill your plate with a variety of colorful vegetables. These provide essential vitamins, minerals,

and fiber. Enjoy them roasted, steamed, stir-fried, or in salads.

5. Healthy Fats: Include small amounts of healthy fats in your dinner. Opt for sources like nuts, seeds, avocado, or extra-virgin olive oil. These fats help enhance flavor and promote satiety.

6. Flavor with Herbs and Spices: Use herbs, spices, and salt-free seasoning blends to add flavor to your dinner without relying on excessive sodium. Experiment with different combinations to create delicious and satisfying meals.

7. Limit Sodium: Be mindful of the sodium content in your dinner choices. Limit the use of high-sodium condiments,

processed meats, and pre-packaged sauces. Instead, opt for homemade seasonings and sauces to control sodium intake.

8. Control Portion Sizes: Pay attention to portion sizes to maintain a balanced dinner. Use measuring cups or a food scale to ensure appropriate servings of grains, proteins, and fats.

9. Hydration: Accompany your dinner with a hydrating beverage, such as water or herbal tea. Limit sugary drinks and alcohol, and opt for healthier options.

7.2 Delicious Dash Diet Dinner Recipes

Here are a few delicious Dash Diet dinner recipes to inspire your evening meals:

1. Baked Salmon with Quinoa and Roasted Vegetables:
    Ingredients:

- 4 ounces salmon fillet

- 1/2 cup cooked quinoa

- Mixed vegetables of your choice (such as broccoli, carrots, and bell peppers)

- 1 tablespoon extra-virgin olive oil

- Salt-free seasoning or herbs of choice

Instructions:

- Preheat the oven to 400°F (200°C).

- Place the salmon fillet on a baking sheet lined with parchment paper.

- Drizzle with olive oil and sprinkle with salt-free seasoning or herbs.

- Roast the salmon in the preheated oven for about 12-15 minutes or until cooked to your desired level of doneness.

- While the salmon is cooking, roast the mixed vegetables tossed in olive oil and salt-free seasoning on a separate baking sheet for about 15-20 minutes or until tender.

- Serve the baked salmon with cooked quinoa and roasted vegetables.

2. Turkey and Vegetable Stir-Fry: Ingredients:

- 4 ounces ground turkey

- 1 cup mixed vegetables (such as broccoli florets, bell peppers, carrots, snap peas)

- 2 cloves garlic, minced

- 2 tablespoons low-sodium soy sauce or tamari

- 1 tablespoon extra-virgin olive oil

- Salt-free seasoning to taste

- Cooked brown rice or quinoa for serving

Instructions:

- Heat olive oil in a skillet or wok over medium-high heat.

- Add minced garlic and sauté for 1 minute until fragrant.

- Add ground turkey and cook until browned and cooked through.

- Add the mixed vegetables and stir-fry until crisp-tender.

- Stir in low-sodium soy sauce or tamari and salt-free seasoning.

- Cook for another 2-3 minutes until everything is heated through.

- Serve the turkey and vegetable stir-fry over cooked brown rice or quinoa.

3. Lentil and Vegetable Curry:
Ingredients:

- 1 cup cooked lentils (green or brown)

- 1 cup mixed vegetables (such as cauliflower, bell peppers, zucchini, and carrots)

- 1 small onion, diced

- 2 cloves garlic, minced

- 1 tablespoon curry powder

- 1 can (14 ounces) diced tomatoes

- 1 cup low-sodium vegetable broth

- 1 tablespoon extra-virgin olive oil

- Salt-free seasoning or herbs of choice

- Cooked brown rice for serving

Instructions:

- Heat olive oil in a large skillet or pot over medium heat.

- Add diced onion and minced garlic, and sauté until onion is translucent.

- Add mixed vegetables and cook until slightly softened.

- Stir in curry powder and salt-free seasoning, and cook for another minute to toast the spices.

- Add cooked lentils, diced tomatoes, and vegetable broth. Simmer for about 10-15 minutes to allow the flavors to meld together.

- Adjust the seasoning if needed.

- Serve the lentil and vegetable curry over cooked brown rice.

4. Grilled Chicken with Quinoa and Steamed Broccoli:
Ingredients:

- 4 ounces grilled chicken breast

- 1/2 cup cooked quinoa

- Steamed broccoli florets

- Lemon juice for seasoning

- 1 teaspoon extra-virgin olive oil

- Salt-free seasoning or herbs of choice

Instructions:

- Season the grilled chicken breast with salt-free seasoning or herbs of choice.

- In a bowl, toss the cooked quinoa with lemon juice, extra-virgin olive oil, and salt-free seasoning.

- Serve the grilled chicken with a side of seasoned quinoa and steamed broccoli.

Feel free to modify these recipes based on your taste preferences and ingredient availability. Adjust portion sizes and ingredient quantities to meet your specific calorie goals and dietary needs. Enjoy these delicious Dash Diet dinner recipes as part of your healthy meal plan.

CHAPTER 8

Snack and Dessert Ideas

8.1 Healthy Dash Diet Snack Options

Snacks can help keep your energy levels stable between meals and prevent overeating. When following the Dash Diet, it's important to choose healthy snack options that align with the guidelines. Here are some healthy Dash Diet snack ideas:

1. Fresh Fruit: Enjoy a variety of fresh fruits, such as apples, bananas, berries, or citrus fruits. They provide essential vitamins, minerals, and fiber.

Pair them with a small handful of nuts or a tablespoon of nut butter for added protein and healthy fats.

2. Vegetable Sticks with Hummus: Slice vegetables like carrots, bell peppers, cucumbers, or celery into sticks and enjoy them with a serving of hummus. This provides a satisfying crunch and a nutrient-packed snack.

3. Greek Yogurt: Choose plain Greek yogurt and top it with fresh berries, a sprinkle of nuts or seeds, and a drizzle of honey or maple syrup for a protein-rich and satisfying snack.

4. Homemade Trail Mix: Create your own trail mix using a combination of unsalted nuts,

seeds, and dried fruits. Mix together almonds, walnuts, pumpkin seeds, sunflower seeds, and dried cranberries or raisins for a nutritious and portable snack.

5. Whole Grain Crackers with Low-Sodium Cheese: Select whole grain crackers and pair them with a small portion of low-sodium cheese. This provides a combination of whole grains, protein, and calcium.

6. Hard-Boiled Eggs: Hard-boiled eggs are a convenient and protein-rich snack option. Sprinkle them with salt-free seasoning or herbs for added flavor.

7. Smoothies: Blend together a combination of fruits, vegetables, low-fat yogurt, and a liquid of your choice, such as water or unsweetened almond milk, to create a nutritious and refreshing snack.

8. Air-Popped Popcorn: Opt for air-popped popcorn instead of traditional buttered popcorn. Season it with herbs, spices, or nutritional yeast for added flavor.

9. Sliced Turkey or Chicken Wraps: Roll up sliced turkey or chicken breast with lettuce, tomato, and other veggies of your choice in a whole grain wrap or lettuce leaf for a protein-rich snack.

10. Edamame: Enjoy a handful of steamed or roasted edamame pods for a protein-packed and fiber-rich snack.

Remember to choose snacks that fit your specific dietary needs and preferences. Pay attention to portion sizes and aim for a balanced combination of macronutrients, including protein, carbohydrates, and healthy fats.

8.2 Tasty Dash Diet Dessert Recipes

While desserts should be consumed in moderation, it's possible to enjoy sweet treats that align with the Dash Diet guidelines. Here are a few tasty Dash Diet dessert recipes:

1. Berry Parfait: Ingredients:

- 1 cup mixed berries (such as strawberries, blueberries, raspberries)

- 1 cup plain Greek yogurt

- 1/4 cup granola (choose a low-sugar and whole grain option)

- 1 tablespoon honey or maple syrup (optional)

Instructions:

- In a glass or bowl, layer half of the mixed berries.

- Top with half of the Greek yogurt.

- Sprinkle with half of the granola.

- Repeat the layers with the remaining ingredients.

- Drizzle with honey or maple syrup if desired.

- Enjoy as a refreshing and nutritious dessert.

2. Dark Chocolate-Dipped Strawberries: Ingredients:

- Fresh strawberries

- Dark chocolate chips (at least 70% cocoa)

- Optional toppings: chopped nuts, shredded coconut, or chia seeds

Instructions:

- Wash and dry the strawberries thoroughly.

- In a microwave-safe bowl, melt the dark chocolate chips in short intervals, stirring in between until smooth.

- Dip each strawberry into the melted dark chocolate, leaving the top part exposed.

- Place the dipped strawberries on a parchment-lined baking sheet.

- Sprinkle with optional toppings, if desired.

- Allow the chocolate to set by refrigerating the strawberries for about 15-20 minutes.

- Enjoy these indulgent yet healthier chocolate-covered strawberries as a satisfying dessert.

3. Banana "Nice Cream":
   Ingredients:

- 2 ripe bananas, peeled and sliced

- 1 tablespoon unsweetened cocoa powder or peanut butter (optional)

- Toppings: chopped nuts, fresh berries, or shredded coconut

Instructions:

- Place the sliced bananas in a single layer on a parchment-lined baking sheet.

- Freeze the banana slices for at least 2 hours or until frozen solid.

- Transfer the frozen banana slices to a blender or food processor.

- Blend until smooth and creamy, stopping to scrape down the sides as needed.

- Add cocoa powder or peanut butter if desired for added flavor.

- Serve the banana "nice cream" immediately with your choice of toppings.

4. Baked Apples with Cinnamon: Ingredients:

- Apples (such as Granny Smith or Honeycrisp)

- Ground cinnamon

- Optional toppings: chopped nuts, raisins, or a drizzle of honey

Instructions:

- Preheat the oven to 375°F (190°C).

- Core the apples, leaving the bottom intact to create a cavity.

- Place the apples on a baking dish lined with parchment paper.

- Sprinkle each apple with ground cinnamon, filling the cavity generously.

- Add optional toppings like chopped nuts or raisins into the cavity if desired.

- Bake the apples for about 25-30 minutes or until tender.

- Serve warm, optionally drizzled with honey.

These dessert recipes can be customized to your taste preferences. Remember to enjoy desserts in moderation as part of a balanced diet.

CHAPTER 9

Meal Prep Tips and Tricks

9.1 Time-Saving Techniques

Meal prep can be made more efficient with time-saving techniques. Here are some tips to help you save time during your Dash Diet meal prep:

1. Plan Ahead: Take some time to plan your meals for the week. This includes deciding on recipes, making a grocery list, and organizing your meal prep schedule. Planning ahead ensures that you have all the necessary ingredients and tools,

reducing last-minute trips to the grocery store.

2. Batch Cooking: As mentioned earlier, batch cooking is a time-saving technique where you cook larger quantities of food at once. This allows you to have pre-cooked components that can be used in multiple meals throughout the week. Cook proteins, whole grains, and roasted vegetables in batches to save time during meal assembly.

3. Use Multitasking: Make use of your kitchen appliances and multitask to save time. For example, while vegetables are roasting in the oven, you can simultaneously cook grains on the stovetop. Look for opportunities to maximize

efficiency and minimize waiting time.

4. Pre-Chop Ingredients: Prepping ingredients in advance can save valuable time during meal prep. Wash, peel, and chop vegetables ahead of time and store them in airtight containers in the refrigerator. This way, they are ready to be used when you need them.

5. Pre-Portion Ingredients: If you have ingredients that need to be portioned, such as snacks or ingredients for grab-and-go meals, pre-portion them in individual containers or resealable bags. This way, you can quickly grab what you need without having to measure or portion them out each time.

6. Use Kitchen Tools and Appliances: Utilize kitchen tools and appliances that can help speed up the meal prep process. Invest in a good quality food processor or blender for chopping, blending, and pureeing ingredients. Use a mandoline slicer or a sharp knife to quickly slice vegetables.

7. Cook Once, Eat Twice: When cooking your main meals, consider making extra portions to be used as leftovers for future meals. This saves time on cooking and allows you to have ready-to-eat meals for busy days.

9.2 Portion Control and Tracking

Portion control and tracking your meals can help you stay on track with the Dash Diet. Here are some tips to help you with portion control and tracking:

1. Use Measuring Tools: Utilize measuring cups, spoons, and a kitchen scale to measure and portion your ingredients accurately. This ensures that you are consuming appropriate serving sizes as recommended by the Dash Diet guidelines.

2. Use Portion-Controlled Containers: Invest in portion-controlled containers that are pre-divided into compartments. These containers can help you visually estimate and control

portion sizes for different food groups.

3. Read Food Labels: Pay attention to food labels to understand portion sizes and nutritional information. Labels provide valuable information on serving sizes, calories, sodium content, and other nutrients. Use this information to make informed choices and track your intake.

4. Use Food Tracking Apps: Consider using food tracking apps or websites to track your meals and monitor your calorie and nutrient intake. These tools allow you to log your meals, set goals, and provide insights into your eating patterns.

5. Keep a Food Diary: Keep a journal or diary to record your meals and snacks. This can help you become more mindful of your food choices and portion sizes. It also serves as a helpful reference when analyzing your eating habits.

6. Practice Mindful Eating: Pay attention to your body's hunger and fullness cues. Eat slowly, savoring each bite, and stop eating when you feel comfortably satisfied. Mindful eating can help prevent overeating and promote a healthier relationship with food.

9.3 Staying Motivated on the Dash Diet

Staying motivated on the Dash Diet can be challenging, but there are strategies to help you stay on track. Here are some tips to stay motivated:

1. Set Realistic Goals: Set achievable and realistic goals that align with the Dash Diet principles. Break down your long-term goals into smaller, manageable milestones. Celebrate your achievements along the way to maintain motivation.

2. Find Accountability Partners: Share your journey with friends, family, or a support group. Having accountability partners can provide encouragement, support, and

help you stay motivated. You can also consider joining online communities or forums focused on the Dash Diet for additional support.

3. Keep Variety in Your Meals: Incorporate a wide variety of foods and flavors into your meals. Experiment with different recipes, spices, and cooking methods to keep your meals interesting and enjoyable. Variety can help prevent boredom and increase satisfaction with your meals.

4. Meal Prep and Plan Ahead: As mentioned earlier, meal prepping and planning can save time and help you stay on track. Knowing that you have healthy meals prepared and ready to go

can reduce the temptation to rely on unhealthy options.

5. Track Your Progress: Keep track of your progress, whether it's through measurements, weight, or other health markers. Seeing tangible results can be motivating and provide reinforcement that your efforts are paying off.

6. Focus on Non-Scale Victories: Instead of solely focusing on the number on the scale, celebrate non-scale victories. These can include increased energy levels, improved sleep quality, reduced cravings, or improved overall well-being. Acknowledge and celebrate these positive changes.

7. Reflect on Your Why: Remind
    yourself of the reasons why you
    chose to follow the Dash Diet.
    Whether it's to improve your
    health, increase energy, or
    manage a specific condition,
    reconnecting with your
    motivations can reignite your
    commitment and motivation.

8. Practice Self-Care: Take care of
    yourself beyond just your diet.
    Prioritize self-care activities
    such as exercise, relaxation
    techniques, quality sleep, and
    stress management. Taking care
    of your overall well-being can
    positively impact your
    motivation and adherence to the
    Dash Diet.